Toronto Physical Examination Series
General Editor: Donald L. Levene, M.D.

CNS

Neurological Examination

Arline McLean, M.D.
Assistant Professor of Neurology,
University of Toronto,
Sunnybrook Medical Centre, Toronto

Collier Macmillan Canada, Ltd.

Copyright © 1980 by Donald L. Levene. All rights re-
served. No part of this book may be reproduced or trans-
mitted in any form by any means, electronic or mechanical,
including photocopying, recording, or by any information
storage and retrieval system, without permission in writing
from the publisher.

Collier Macmillan Canada, Ltd.
1125B Leslie Street, Don Mills, Ontario M3C 2K2

ISBN 02-991320-9

Design: Michael van Elsen

Illustrations by Margot MacKay, B.S., Department of Art
as Applied to Medicine, University of Toronto

    2 3 4 5 6 84 83 82 81
Printed and bound in Canada.

Canadian Cataloguing in Publication Data

McLean, A. (Arline), 1939 –
    C.N.S. : neurological examination

(Toronto physical examination series)

ISBN 0-02-991320-9

1. Neurologic examination – Handbooks, manuals, etc.
I. Title.   II. Title: Neurological examination.
III. Series.

RC348.M34   616.8′0475   C81-094036-1

Contents

Mental State

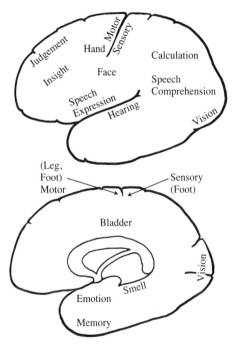

The mental state is one of the many functions of the brain. Different mental functions are subserved by different areas of the brain. Testing the mental state is thus a test of the functions of various parts of the brain.

Much of the mental state can be assessed while taking the history. The following features should be noted.

1. Level of consciousness – alert, drowsy, stuporous, semi-comatose, comatose

2. Behaviour and emotion

3. Trend of thought – orderly, concise, tangential, confused, irrelevant, illusions, delusions, hallucinations, comprehension, and judgement

4. Intellectual function – orientation to time, person and place; general knowledge; ability to abstract – proverbs; calculation – ask the patient to do serial subtractions: 100-7 or 20-3; memory – immediate memory: repetition of numbers forward and backward or immediate recall of a short story; recent memory: recall of specific objects, names, address (patient told he is expected to remember these when given them) or recall of events earlier in the day; content of recent meals; remote memory: recall of past events

5. Language functions – verbal, written, visual, and auditory. If a dysphasia is present you should be able to place it in one of three main categories: receptive, expressive, or receptive-expressive dysphasia

6. spatial orientation; body image, sensory inattention; agnosias, apraxias

Cranial Nerve I

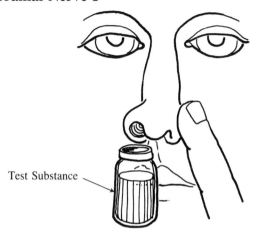

Test Substance

Test each naris separately, with the other occluded. Have the patient gently sniff a non-irritating volatile substance such as oil of cloves or lemon. Aromatic substances such as coffee may also be used. Ask the patient if he can perceive and identify the test substance; compare the two nares.

Unilateral anosmia:
blocked naris
sphenoid ridge or
   olfactory groove
      meningioma
unilateral ethmoiditis

Bilateral anosmia:
U.R.I.
heavy smoker
post head injury
pituitary lesions
hysteria

Cranial Nerve 2: Visual Fields

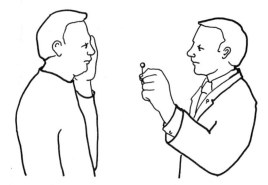

First determine the visual acuity of each eye with the Snellen chart, or, if necessary, by counting fingers. Have the patient sit directly opposite you, cover one eye and fix his other eye on your directly opposite eye, e.g., his right eye on your left eye. Map each field separately using a 3 mm white test object and compare with your own ('normal'). Start from the periphery and move the test object into the field of vision keeping it half way between you and the patient. Do at least 4 radii for each eye.

If the patient wears glasses, test him with glasses on. If the patient's visual acuity is very poor or co-operation is limited, gross hand movements may be used.

Bilateral stimulation of the visual fields tests for visual inattention.

Cranial Nerve 2: Pathway and Typical Field Defects

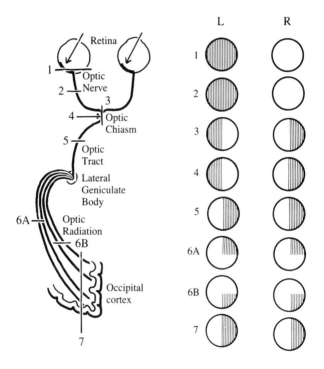

L   R

1. Retina
   Optic Nerve
2. Optic Nerve
3. Optic Chiasm
4. Optic Chiasm
5. Optic Tract
   Lateral Geniculate Body
6A. Optic Radiation
6B.
   Occipital cortex
7.

Cranial Nerve 2: Typical Field Defects

1. Unilateral field loss:
   retinal hemorrhage, venous thrombosis

2. Unilateral field loss:
   optic nerve glioma, optic neuritis
   sphenoid ridge meningioma

3. Bitemporal heteronymous hemianopia:
   tumor (pituitary, craniopharyngioma), trauma

4. Bitemporal hemianopia or blindness of the ipsilateral
   eye with temporal hemianopia of the contralateral
   eye:
   dilated internal carotid
   suprasellar meningioma

5. Homonymous hemianopia (contralateral):
   vascular (infarct)
   compressive (tumor, abscess, SDH)

6. Contralateral homonymous defects – partial to com-
   plete hemianopias:
   vascular (infarct, hemorrhage)
   S.O.L. – tumor, abscess

7. Unilateral lesion – homonymous field defects:
   hemianopic, quadrantic defects with sparing of cen-
   tral vision, e.g., in post-cerebral artery occlusion.

Funduscopic Examinations

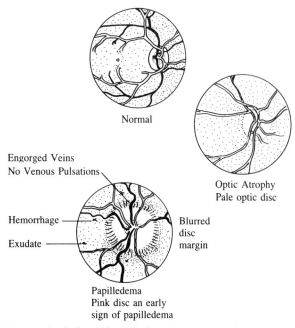

Normal

Optic Atrophy
Pale optic disc

Engorged Veins
No Venous Pulsations

Hemorrhage

Exudate

Blurred
disc
margin

Papilledema
Pink disc an early
sign of papilledema

Observe both fundi in a darkened room; avoid mydriatics.
Have the patient fix his eyes on a distant object.
Correct for your own refractive error if present.
Examine the disc, vessels, macula, retina.

Cranial Nerves 3, 4, 6

Direction of movement of the eyeball by the extra ocular muscles

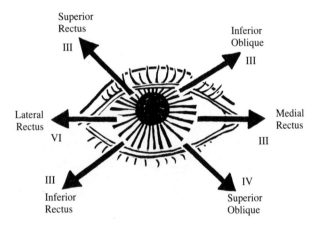

Have the patient follow a light as you move it in each direction of gaze. If he notes diplopia, have him tell you the orientation of the image, and by covering the eyes alternately, determine which image is the false one. (It is the outside image in the direction of gaze of the paretic muscle.) Note also the lids (ptosis or lid retraction) and position of the eyes.

12

Examination of Pupils

Observe size, shape, symmetry, and reflexes.

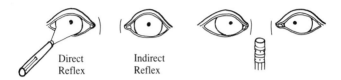

Direct Reflex   Indirect Reflex

Light Reflexes
Have the patient look at a distant object. Flash a light into one eye. Both pupils should constrict.

Accommodation-Convergence Reflex
Both pupils constrict when the patient looks from a distant object to a near object, e.g., a pencil 10 cm away.

Unilateral fixed dilated pupil – ipsilateral C.N. 3 paralysis. Useful in localizing pathology to the ipsilateral hemisphere in a comatose patient.
Pin point fixed pupils in a comatose patient suggest a brainstem lesion.
Argyll-Robertson pupils – small irregular pupils, nonreactive to light but react to accommodation convergence. Seen in syphilis.

Cranial Nerve 5: Sensation

Light touch, pain – see Sensory Examination

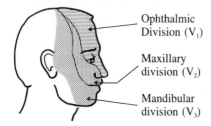

Ophthalmic Division (V_1)

Maxillary division (V_2)

Mandibular division (V_3)

Corneal reflex

Wisp of cotton

Have the patient look away and approach from the side to avoid a blink from a visual response

Positive response – blinking of the ipsilateral eye (direct corneal reflex) and of the contralateral eye (consensual corneal reflex):

If the sensory arc is intact but not the motor, blinking of the contralateral eye only occurs.

If the sensory arc is not intact neither eye blinks; however if the motor arc is intact when the sensory is not, blinking will occur with stimulation of the contralateral eye.

Cranial Nerve 5: Motor

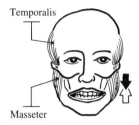

Masseter and temporalis muscles:
Elevate the mandible.
To test, have the patient clench his jaws and palpate the contracting masseter and temporalis muscles.

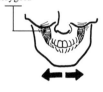

Pterygoid muscles:
Deviate the mandible from side to side; depress and protrude the mandible especially the external pterygoids.
If they are paralyzed, the jaw deviates to the side of the paralyzed muscle and the involved nerve.

Jaw jerk – tap your finger, which is placed on the middle of the patient's chin (mouth slightly open). Minimal jaw elevation is normal; brisk jaw elevation suggests a supranuclear lesion.

Cranial Nerve 7

1. Motor: facial muscles, including platysma
   Have the patient: frown, smile, whistle, grimace,
   squeeze his eyes shut while the examiner tries to force
   them open.

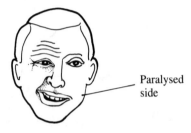

Paralysed
side

UMN - only the lower half of the face is weak or para-
       lyzed
     - the paralysis is contralateral to the lesion

LMN - upper and lower facial weakness; as above

2. Sensory: Taste to the anterior ⅔ of the tongue
   Test sweet, sour, bitter, and salt, using colourless
   solutions. With the patient's eyes closed, apply the
   solution with a cotton swab or dropper to each side
   separately. Do not allow the patient to withdraw his
   tongue into his mouth and therefore stimulate the
   uninvolved side.

3. Autonomic: lacrimation and salivation

Cranial Nerve 8: Acoustic

Normal – loud whisper audible at 2m; watch ticking audible next to external auditory meatus. To mask one ear while testing the other, have the patient hold a piece of paper beside one ear and scratch the paper.

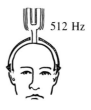

512 Hz

Rinne test
Place the handle of a tuning fork on the mastoid process; when the patient no longer perceives the sound, place the fork next to the ear; compare with yourself.

Rinne positive (air > bone) normal or sensorineural loss
Rinne negative (air < bone) conductive loss (middle ear disease)

Weber test
Place the handle of a vibrating tuning fork on the vertex of the skull. Sound should be heard equally in both ears in the normal. Lateralization away from the affected side (towards the normal side) occurs in unilateral sensorineural loss.

Cranial Nerve 8: Vestibular

Nystagmus

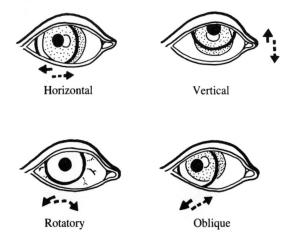

Have the patient look in all directions of gaze and observe each eye for nystagmus.

Record: the direction of the quick phase
the direction in which nystagmus is maximal

Note: Minimal, non-sustained horizontal jerk nystagmus observed with the adducting eye deviated beyond the inner canthus may be physiological.

Cranial Nerves 9 and 10

Pharyngeal pain fibres are supplied by C.N. 9 while tactile sensation and motor innervation are supplied by C.N. 10.

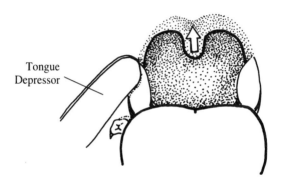

Test each side of the pharynx and soft palate by stimulating with a tongue depressor. Palatal and pharyngeal reflexes are lost with C.N. 9 impairment. With C.N. 10 impairment pharyngeal paresis occurs with nasal speech, hoarse voice, and difficulty in swallowing.

C.N. 9 supplies taste to the posterior ⅓ of the tongue, but it is difficult to test. So also is the stylopharyngeus muscle that C.N. 9 innervates.

Parasympathetic C.N. 9 innervates the inferior salivary nucleus.

Cranial Nerve 11

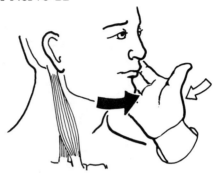

The patient laterally rotates his head against resistance.

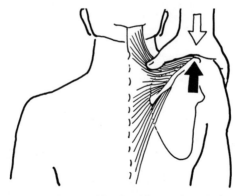

The patient elevates his shoulder against resistance.

Cranial Nerve 12

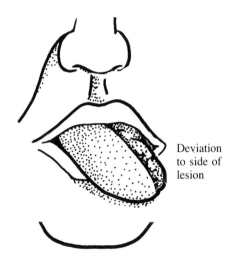

Deviation to side of lesion

Observe the tongue at rest for shape, position, fasiculations, wasting. Percuss for myotonia. Have the patient move the tongue rapidly from side to side, push out the cheek against force, protrude the tongue observing for deviation from the midline. Unilateral 12th nerve palsy causes deviation of the protruded tongue to the side of the lesion. In bilateral 12th nerve palsy the patient cannot protrude his tongue.

Motor Examination: General Comments

Distribution of wasting:
focal – i.e., one limb; nerve root distribution or peripheral nerve distribution
proximal – myopathy vs. distal – peripheral neuropathy
facial (myopathy)

Fasciculations:
don't forget the tongue (ALS)
fasciculations in the absence of wasting or weakness and limited to the calves – benign

Tone: ↑ in UMN lesions
↓ in LMN lesions, cerebellar disease
- determine the distribution of changes in tone, e.g., the arm and leg on one side, etc.

Power loss:
peripheral nerve distribution, e.g., median nerve
nerve root distribution
proximal muscles vs. distal
spinal cord level
monoplegia
hemiplegia, quadriplegia, ± facial involvement

Palpate for consistency and tenderness.
Percuss for myotonia.

Muscle Bulk

Hypertrophy	Normal	Atrophy

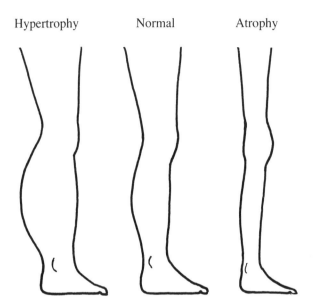

Duchenne muscular
dystrophy
'Excessive use'

- occurs in LMN
  disorders
- AHC
- nerve root
- neuropathy
- myopathy

Muscle Tone

With the patient relaxed, test resistance to passive flexion of the elbow, knee, wrist.

Normally there is smooth minimal passive resistance

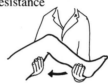

Lead-pipe rigidity

Steady, marked increase in tone through full range of movement

Clasp knife phenomenon

Initial marked increase in tone followed by sudden release

Cogwheel rigidity

Intermittent rachet-like increase in tone

Muscle Power

Position the patient for optimum function of the muscle being tested. The patient actively resists force initiated by the examiner. The tested muscle can usually be seen and palpated. Use MRC grading of strength 0 to 5 (normal).

Supraspinatus
Suprascapular nerve
C5, 6 segments

Supraspinatus
1st 20°
Deltoid
20-90°

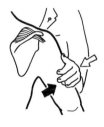

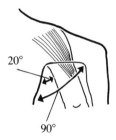

20°

90°

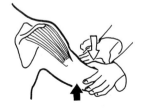

Deltoid
Axillary nerve C5, 6
segments

Muscle Power 1

Pectoralis major

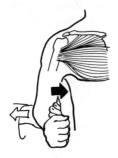

Infraspinatus

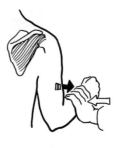

Medial and lateral pectoral nerves C5, 6, <u>7</u>, <u>8</u>, T1 segments

Suprascapular nerve C<u>5</u>, 6 segments

Biceps

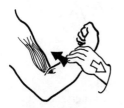

Brachioradialis

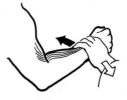

Musculocutaneous nerve C<u>5</u>, <u>6</u> segments

Radial nerve C<u>5</u>, <u>6</u> segments

Muscle Power 2

Triceps

Radial nerve C6, _7_, _8_ segments

Wrist extension

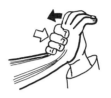

Radial nerve C_6_, _7_, 8 segments. Extensor carpi radialis longus and ulnaris.

Extensor digitorum

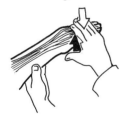

Radial nerve C_7_, 8 segments

Wrist flexion

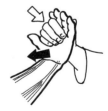

Median nerve C_6_, _7_, 8 segments (flexor carpi radialis). Ulnar nerve C7, _8_, T1 segments flexor carpi ulnaris

Muscle Power 3

Hand grip

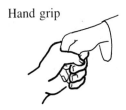

Median nerve (flexor digitorum sublimus and profundus)
Ulnar nerve (flexor digitorum profundus) C7, 8, T1 segments

Abductor pollicus brevis

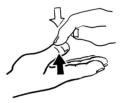

Median nerve
C8, T1 segments

Abductor digiti minimi

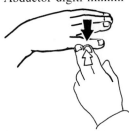

Ulnar nerve C8, T1 segments

1st dorsal interosseus

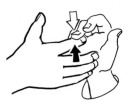

Ulnar nerve, C8, T1 segments

Iliopsoas

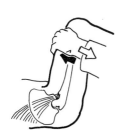

Femoral nerve, lumbar plexus L1, <u>2</u>, <u>3</u>, 4 segments

Hip adductors

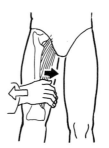

Obdurator nerve L<u>2</u>, <u>3</u>, 4, segments

Hip abductors

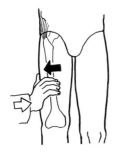

Superior gluteal nerve <u>L4</u>, <u>5</u>, <u>S1</u> segments

Gluteus maximus

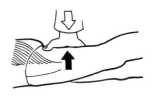

Inferior gluteal nerve <u>L5</u>, <u>S1</u>, 2 segments

Quadriceps femoris

Hamstrings

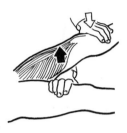

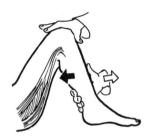

Femoral nerve
L2, <u>3</u>, <u>4</u> segments

Sciatic nerve
L4, <u>5</u>, <u>S1</u>, 2 segments

Tibialis anterior

Gastrocnemius, soleus

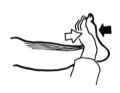

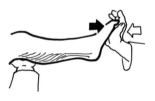

Deep peroneal nerve
<u>L4</u>, 5, S1 segments

Tibial nerve
L5, <u>S1</u>, <u>2</u> segments

Peronei

Tibialis posterior

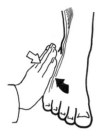

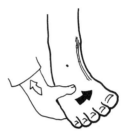

Superficial peroneal nerve
L4, 5, S1 segments

Posterior tibial nerve L5,
S1 segments

Extensor hallucus longus

Extensor digitorum brevis

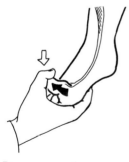

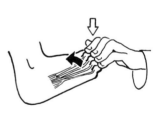

Deep peroneal nerve
(L4), 5, S1 segments

Deep peroneal nerve
L4, 5, S1 segments

Deep Tendon Reflexes: Upper Limbs

The patient must be relaxed and properly positioned. Record as 0 (absent) to + + + + (pathologically brisk) + + = normal

Biceps

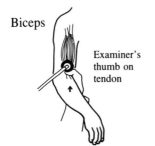

Examiner's thumb on tendon

Musculocutaneous nerve C_5_, 6

Triceps

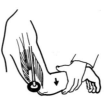

Radial nerve C6, _7_, 8

Supinator

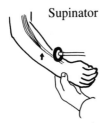

Radial nerve C5, _6_

Finger jerk

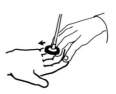

Median and ulnar nerves C7, _8_

Deep Tendon Reflexes: Lower Limbs

Reinforcement (the patient clasps his hands tightly together) should be used if these reflexes appear to be absent.

Knee Jerk

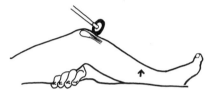

Femoral nerve L3, _4_   Ankle jerk

Medial hamstrings jerk

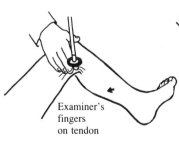

Examiner's
fingers
on tendon

Sciatic nerve L5, S1   Sciatic nerve S1, 2

Superficial Reflexes

Abdominal reflexes

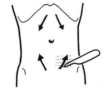

Patient relaxed

Stroke the abdomen lightly with a blunt object. Response is ipsilateral contraction of abdominal muscles.

Babinsky response

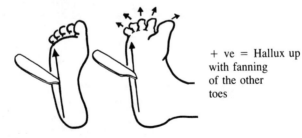

+ ve = Hallux up
with fanning
of the other
toes

With the patient relaxed, stroke the lateral side of the sole with a sharp instrument (key, split tongue depressor). Babinski response is positive in UMN lesions.

Clonus

The patient must be relaxed.

Ankle clonus

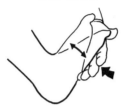

The examiner briskly dorsiflexes the ankle and observes and feels the rapid oscillations of clonus.

Patellar clonus

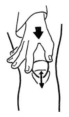

Clasp the patella between the thumb and fingers; briskly push the patella inferiorly. Feel for the oscillation of clonus.

Sensory Examination: General Comments

Determine:

1. if a loss is 'hemisensory' and if there is facial involvement either ipsilateral or contralateral to limb involvement
2. if a loss is in a segmental distribution and if it is single (e.g., root lesion), multiple, or if there is a level as in a spinal cord lesion
3. if a loss is in a peripheral nerve distribution and if it is:
   single as in mononeuropathy, e.g., ulnar, median, etc.
   multiple discrete nerve involvement as in mononeuritis multiplex, diabetes mellitus, or vasculitis
   peripheral neuropathy with stocking-glove loss as in diabetic, alcoholic, uremic, or carcinomatous neuropathies
4. if there is an heredity factor

Palpate peripheral nerves for enlargement, tenderness. Test the sensory function of the cortex by the 2 point discrimination, sensory localization, and object recognition tests. Note that primary sensory modalities (pain, temperature, etc.) must be intact for these tests.

N.B. Always start testing from the area of least sensation and dilineate its extent by working out radially from it.

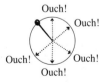

Segmental and Peripheral Nerve Sensory Distributions

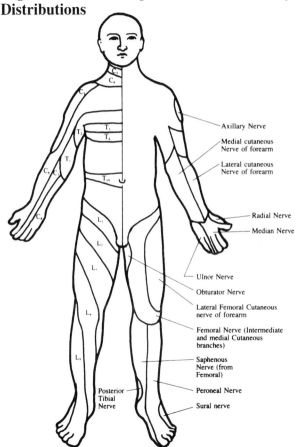

Pain and Temperature

Temperature

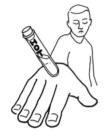

Test tube of hot or cold water (not hot enough to burn!)

Use tubes of hot and cold water or the cold metal of a tuning fork and the warmth of a finger as *poor* substitutes. Determine if the patient (eyes closed) can distinguish between hot and cold.

Superficial pain

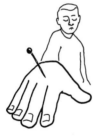

Don't draw blood!

Use light, even, stimuli

Deep pain
Apply pressure over a tendon (e.g., Achilles), or a nerve (e.g., supraorbital). Deep pain is classically lost in Tabes dorsalis.

Pathway for Pain and Temperature

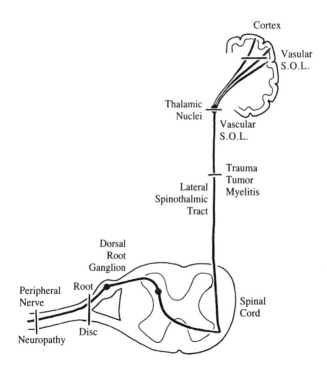

Cortex

Vasular
S.O.L.

Thalamic
Nuclei

Vascular
S.O.L.

Trauma
Tumor
Myelitis

Lateral
Spinothalmic
Tract

Dorsal
Root
Ganglion

Peripheral
Nerve

Root

Disc

Neuropathy

Spinal
Cord

Light Touch

Use a wisp of cotton and touch lightly, don't stroke (tickle). The patient (eyes closed) tells the examiner each time he feels a light touch.

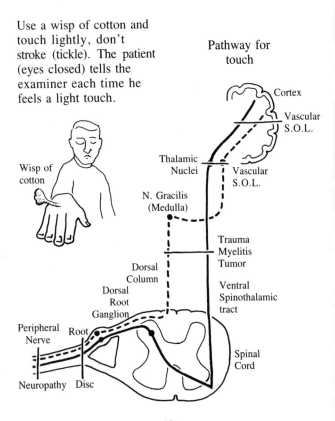

Pathway for touch

Cortex

Vascular S.O.L.

Thalamic Nuclei

Vascular S.O.L.

N. Gracilis (Medulla)

Trauma
Myelitis
Tumor

Wisp of cotton

Ventral Spinothalamic tract

Dorsal Column

Dorsal Root Ganglion

Peripheral Nerve

Root

Spinal Cord

Neuropathy Disc

Position and Vibration Sense

Vibration

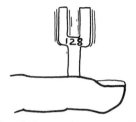

Place the tuning fork over bony prominences beginning with the fingers and great toe. Test the patient's threshold to vibration by allowing the vibrations to decrease until the patient no longer feels it; if absent or decreased distally, determine the proximal level where it is normal.

Position

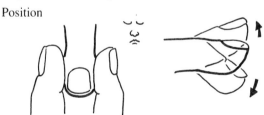

Move the digit up or down. The patient (eyes closed) tells the examiner which direction he thinks his digit (finger, big toe) was moved with each excursion. Fine movements should be detectable. If not, determine the degree and level of impairment.

Pathway for Position and Vibration Senses

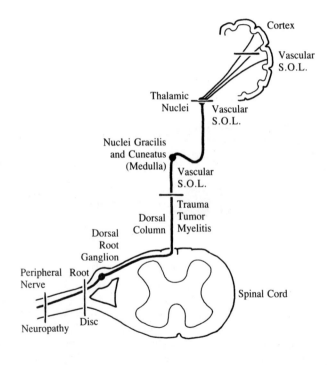

Cortex

Vascular S.O.L.

Thalamic Nuclei

Vascular S.O.L.

Nuclei Gracilis and Cuneatus (Medulla)

Vascular S.O.L.

Trauma Tumor Myelitis

Dorsal Column

Dorsal Root Ganglion

Peripheral Nerve

Root

Neuropathy

Disc

Spinal Cord

Romberg

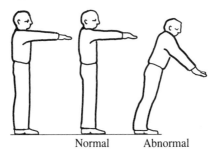

Normal   Abnormal

The patient stands with his feet together and then closes his eyes. Stand close to the patient (to catch him if he falls) but do not touch him.

Gait and Stance

Observe the patient standing, feet together; note steadiness (truncal ataxia), postural abnormalities. Observe the patient walking, turning quickly, doing tandem gait. Observe limps, spasticity, unsteadiness, staggering, etc.

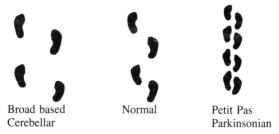

Broad based   Normal   Petit Pas
Cerebellar   Parkinsonian

Cerebellar Testing

Finger – nose

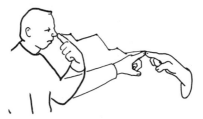

The patient with open eyes touches alternately his nose and the examiner's finger. Normally the action should be smooth and accurate. Side to side deviation and over shoot is abnormal.

Heel – shin

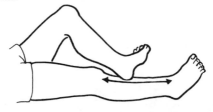

Have the patient slide his heel down his shin; normally the action is smooth and accurate. Side to side deviation is abnormal. Make allowances if weakness is present.

Rapid alternating movements

Alternate supination – pronation of hand

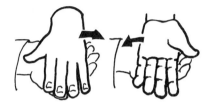

Successive finger-thumb apposition

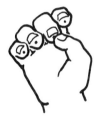

Finger-tapping   Toe-tapping

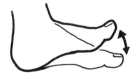

Meningeal Irritation

Nuchal rigidity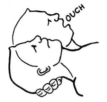

Normal - no resistance in forward flexion
Abnormal - resistance to passive neck flexion

Watch: Severe DDD may give the impression of resistance, but there will also be limitation of rotation and lateral flexion.

Kernig's sign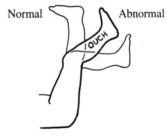

With the hip flexed, attempt to passively extend the knee. If extension is limited and there is pain and spasm of the hamstrings muscles, the sign is positive. This is present in lumbar root irritation as well.

Lasegue's Sign

Lumbar nerve root irritation

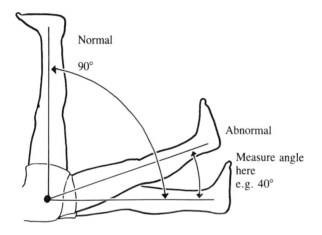

The examiner passively flexes the patient's hip, with the knee extended.

Normal - the leg should be flexed to 90° with minimal if any discomfort - there may be some tightening of the hamstrings muscles but it should not be painful.
Abnormal - passive straight leg raising is limited. May be present bilaterally in meningeal irritation.

Pulses, Bruits, and Blood Pressure

Listen for bruits

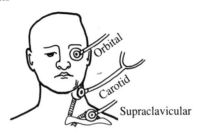

Feel for pulses

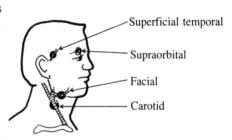

Blood pressure
Brachial blood pressure should be measured in both arms. A significantly lower pressure in one arm suggests occlusive disease in the subclavian artery on that side.

Don't forget to palpate the scalp and skull and examine spinal movements. Note movement disorders.